Fernanda Martin Catarucci

Essays on Metaphysical Self-Healing

Fernanda Martin Catarucci

Essays on Metaphysical Self-Healing

What science has pointed out about the body's ability to heal itself

ScienciaScripts

Imprint

Cover image: Provided by the author

This book is a translation from the original published under ISBN 978-3-330-75684-7.

Publisher:
Sciencia Scripts
is a trademark of
Dodo Books Indian Ocean Ltd. and OmniScriptum S.R.L publishing group

120 High Road, East Finchley, London, N2 9ED, United Kingdom
Str. Armeneasca 28/1, office 1, Chisinau MD-2012, Republic of Moldova, Europe
Printed at: see last page
ISBN: 978-620-8-06026-8

I dedicate this work to all beings who have accepted the challenge of returning to themselves.

Thanks

This work is the result of my dissertation, defended at the Department of Public Health of the Botucatu-UNESP Faculty of Medicine, which sought to gather and synthesize academic production on metaphysical self-healing in national and international databases.

I would like to thank those who participated directly in my master's journey: Marina Cruz, Ivan Guerrini, Regina Stella Spagnuolo, Ione Morita, Karina Pavao and Alberto Peribanez Gonzalez.

And also the people who are supporting this work, who feed my soul with their presence: my parents, siblings, partner, friends, teachers, students and patients. It has been a pleasure to share this project and life with all of you.

Namaste

"Your natural forms, the ones inside you, will be the ones that cure your illnesses"

Hippocrates

SUMMARY

Chapter 1 12

Chapter 2 16

Chapter 3 21

Preface

I first came into contact with this subject while studying physiotherapy, when my brother became very ill. Despite having access to the best doctors and hospitals, it was an acupuncturist who saved his life by reversing a serious process of malnutrition caused by autoimmune pathology.

At that moment my universe expanded, I realized that there was much more to the patient's health/disease process. What I was being taught at university wasn't the only truth. I began to study integrative and complementary practices, starting with Chinese medicine, which is a great passion of mine.

After graduating, I set up a clinic and was invited to work at an acupuncture school, coordinating outpatient clinics and teaching classes. After ten years of practice, and despite the fact that the results were better than those of conventional physiotherapy alone, I still had concerns about relapses and limiting results with chronic illnesses.

Other work proposals related to complementary practices emerged. I studied ayurveda, naturopathy and shamanism, and noticed a common thread in relation to pathophysiology and treatments: both were based on strengthening the biological terrain.

During this same period, I became ill and also didn't respond to conventional treatments. I sought holistic treatments, which gave me better results, but although they were more spontaneous, I still had very painful crises.

I decided to apply the knowledge I had studied. I started meditating, having more contact with nature and improved my diet. The response was impressive. I learned to understand my body's signals and master my "sickness" process. Healing manifested itself not only in my body, but in my life, because these are fields that are not dissociated.

Sharing this knowledge with my patients and students, and realizing that they too have been cured, and that other people are writing and researching about it is what gave me the strength to talk about these experiences in my courses and write my dissertation.

In my master's work, I searched for articles published on self-healing between 2001 and 2011 in national and international scientific journals. I selected and discussed eighty-nine papers, trying to bridge the gap between science and ancient health knowledge.

This research is presented to society through this publication, allowing for reflection and the possibility of contact with this ancient knowledge, stored in each of us, which awaits the moment we decide to connect to it.

INTRODUCED

The World Health Organization (WHO) has recognized the widespread use of Traditional Medicines (TM) in developing countries and the growing use of Complementary and Alternative Medicine (CAM) in developed countries.

The Brazilian Ministry of Health (MoH), in response to the need to find out about experiences that have already been developed in the public health system, carried out a "National Diagnostic", which showed the structure of some of these practices in 232 municipalities, including 19 capitals. As a result of this survey, the National Policy for Integrative and Complementary Practices (PNPIC) in the Unified Health System (SUS) was approved in 2006.

The PNPIC includes complex medical systems and therapeutic resources, which involve approaches that seek to stimulate the natural mechanisms of disease prevention and health recovery, with an emphasis on welcoming listening, the development of the therapeutic bond and the integration of the human being with the environment and society.

The growing popularity of MCA is a reflection of the changing needs and values of modern society in general, stemming from an increase in the prevalence of chronic illnesses, greater access to information, a desire for more control and freedom in relation to one's own health care, an increased sense of designation of a better quality of life, a decline in the belief that conventional medicine will have greater relevance in the treatment of a personal illness and an increased interest in spirituality, self-fulfillment and personal growth.

The various approaches covered in the field of MCA take a broad view of the health-disease process and the overall promotion of human care, especially self-care. It encompasses an extensive variety of therapeutic and diagnostic modalities.

According to the classification adopted by the National Center for Complementary and Alternative Medicine (NCCAM), these practices can be divided into the following categories: a) complete medical systems (includes homeopathy, naturopathy and traditional medicines such as Chinese and Ayurvedic); b) mind-body interventions (includes meditation and prayer); c) biology-based therapies (includes orthomolecular therapy and phytotherapy); d) body manipulation methods (includes chiropractic, osteopathy and massage); e) energy therapies (includes qi gong, reiki and magnetotherapy).

These practices don't just eliminate symptoms, as is the case with chemical drugs or surgical interventions. Their methods stimulate the body's immune system to eliminate toxins or fight pathogens more easily on its own.

The philosophies of these techniques are based on the principle of self-healing, the aim of which is to stimulate health before trying to cure the illness, as it is believed that the stimuli and specific causes of the illness are only effective when the body allows them to be. Therefore, it is not enough to eliminate the symptoms, but it is necessary to understand the reasons that brought about the imbalance, so that a cure can really be established.

In this way it is possible to differentiate the term self-healing according to its proposed intervention. Robb (2003) classified them into five categories: "Synthetic Self-Healing" (referring to a polymer that repairs materials used in the body, such as prostheses), "Cybernetic Healing" (a device that restores an incorrect operation in the body, without human intervention) and "Biophysical Self-Healing" (which is carried out inside the body's cells, as occurs with embryonic cells).

These first three categories believe that the body's ability to heal lies only in eradicating the symptoms of the illness, and many therapists of the MCA modalities operate with the same Western thinking, believing that they promote healing by using their alternative techniques to reduce or eliminate the patient's complaints.

This may explain why more than 30% of people who visit an alternative medicine practitioner say they feel "very unhappy" with the treatments they receive.

However, the other two categories broaden this definition. The group called "Self-Help" includes tools designed to instruct on techniques for healing or improving oneself (such as books, courses and creams). And in the last modality, in which this work is centered, "Metaphysical Self-Healing" explains that our intuitive aspect would know how to exist or return to harmony, and illness would only be an expression of an imbalance in our lives, orienting it towards a more favorable and satisfactory direction.

In this way, metaphysical self-healing is identified as a natural, unique and individual process, which occurs from within, restoring balance to systems, and enabling self-diagnosis and repair without conscious effort. An active process in which patients take responsibility for their own health.

The inner dialogue technique, suggested by Clark (1981) as a self-healing approach, consists of relaxation exercises that allow for a meditative state in which the patient consults their inner counselor, who knows all the reasons for the imbalances and can help in the rebalancing process.

A study carried out on a health insurance population in the United States lasted 11 years and compared 2,000 people who practiced meditation with 600,000 who didn't, and found a 63% reduction in healthcare costs, 11.4 times fewer hospital admissions for cardiovascular disease, 3.3 times fewer for cancer and 6.7 times fewer for mental disorders and substance abuse in those who practiced meditation.

The use of MCA can help reduce medical costs by preventing and treating illnesses, as well as providing more humanized care that respects patients' philosophies and beliefs.

Recent studies believe that relying on this internal force, rather than the effects of drugs, would be useful in treating illnesses, as it produces natural compensatory mechanisms.

It would be an innate ability, often dismissed in studies as a placebo effect, as something that must be controlled and eliminated.

The connection to this inner force can be achieved through natural methods that help to rebalance the body. These are autonomous activities that benefit health, such as massage, stretching, breathing, visualization, meditation, relaxation, imagination, hypnosis, yoga, tai chi, energy touch therapies, acupressure, reflexology, healing prayer, shamanism, sex and laughter.

But it's not enough to take care of our minds; we must also try to keep our biological terrain, which are our cells, clean and healthy, because this is the only way we can prevent harmless microscopic beings that live in symbiosis within us from being replaced by multi-resistant parasitic microbes.

In this sense, we must avoid external factors and influences that damage the balance of health, as they exert forces that make it difficult for the body to return to a state of harmony.

Reduced physical exertion, stress, thermal variations (air conditioning and low exposure to sunlight) and industrialized food, which characterize modern life, are factors that can result in these systemic dysfunctions.

In recent decades, it has become important to take care of life in such a way as to reduce vulnerability to illness and the chances of it producing disability, chronic suffering and premature death.

In the SUS, the National Health Promotion Policy (PNPS) is a strategy to take up the possibility of focusing on these aspects that determine the health-disease process, broadening the ways of intervening in health.

A cooperative exchange between the systems, which understands that therapeutic procedures can combine conventional and alternative techniques and medicines without a common theoretical basis, can help redefine the paradigm of Western medicine.

1. The Voice of Users of Self-Healing Practices

Research aimed at characterizing users of self-healing practices has concluded that women (62%) who are older, better educated and in poorer health conditions are more likely to use Traditional Medicine and Complementary and Alternative Medicine.

With regard to the type of practice, there is a significant number of users, especially when prayer, which is the most cited, is included as one of these therapies. The other most cited practices are vitamins, supplements, diet therapy, meditation, massage and music therapy.

Religious and non-religious patients with rheumatoid arthritis (RA) were interviewed and it was observed that positive coping scores in relation to the pathology were related to religious people, who coped better with the emotional stress caused by the pathology.

The same was observed with cancer patients, where 68.5% reported having prayed for their own health and 72% reported their state of health as "good" or "better".

But not all research classifies prayer as complementary or alternative medicine. Studies have shown that when all types of practice are included, i.e. those with an alternative therapist or that are self-performed by the user (such as prayer), the percentage of practitioners reaches 98%. However, when attributing the use of complementary and alternative medicine to the presence of a therapist, this proportion is reduced to just 20% of users.

Another Brazilian study shows a prevalence of 9% in the use of complementary and alternative medicines when considering only those that involve costs and therefore the presence of a therapist (homeopathy, acupuncture, chiropractic, orthomolecular medicine, relaxation/meditation techniques and massage); and 70% when including all therapies, such as prayer.

The National Policy on Integrative and Complementary Practices was a great achievement in terms of the need to get to know, support, incorporate and implement experiences that have already been developed in the public network of many municipalities and states.

The study of the situational diagnosis of integrative and complementary practices in the SUS observed the existence of some of these practices in 26 states of the Federation, with a concentration in the states of the southeast region.

This number could be much higher, as it is a variable that depends on the classification of integrative and complementary practices by the Department of Primary Care and the state and municipal departments of the country that answered the situational diagnosis questionnaire. This data may even explain the concentration of the southeast region in the SUS situational diagnosis.

The results of the situational diagnosis in the SUS also showed that in terms of frequency, Reiki and Lian Gong are predominant, followed by Phytotherapy, Homeopathy and Acupuncture, and that the actions are preferably inserted in Basic Care - Family Health.

As a result, the strategy for drawing up this policy was to form sub-working groups, represented by the Brazilian Associations of Phytotherapy, Homeopathy, Acupuncture and Anthroposophical Medicine.

We observed that although Reiki (a technique based on chakra theory) and Lian Gong (a practice that belongs to Chinese Medicine theory) were the most cited practices in the SUS situational diagnosis, they had no representatives in the drafting of the national policy.

The sub-groups represented by the Brazilian Associations of Phytotherapy, Homeopathy, Acupuncture and Anthroposophical Medicine have created general guidelines that cover all integrative and complementary practices, but the description of the implementation of these guidelines has only been specified for the areas represented by these sub-groups. In practice, this could represent more support for the implementation of and research into the practices encompassed by these groups.

In this way, we have opened up options for alternative interventions, the advantages of which are treatments with fewer side effects and lower costs compared to allopathic medicine, but which maintain the patient's dependence on a therapist in order to intervene in their illness process, since the techniques proposed in the guidelines insist on acting like conventional medicine, i.e. they seek to rebalance the patient's disharmony, but without understanding the causal factor of the illness, thus keeping the user passive in this process.

Another issue raised by the researchers was the significant number of alternative medicines that could interact negatively with allopathic medication. This reality is exacerbated by the fact that most studies show that patients do not discuss the use of these therapies with their healthcare team.

When patients were asked about their decision not to talk to their doctors, the reasons given were: "because it wasn't important", "the doctor wouldn't be interested" and "the doctor doesn't know about complementary and alternative medicines".

One study showed that the strong scientific support of a technique for a particular pathology did not interfere with the choice of practice. Mind-body therapies were used infrequently for chronic pain (20%), insomnia (13%), by less than 20% of patients with heart disease, headaches, sore throats or cancer. These are conditions in which clinical consensus has concluded that mind-body therapies are effective.

In most of the articles, the incentive and information to start using these practices came from a friend or relative, i.e. the dissemination of the results of these methods comes from personal experiences shared in heterogeneous social groups.

The search for this support has led many patients to turn to the internet. Cancer patients have found in this option elements that provide a way of living with a chronic illness instead of simply accepting the "death sentence".

The insufficient care provided to patients in conventional medicine appears to be one of the reasons for choosing to use CAM, but it is not the only one. Patients with chronic illnesses cited that the main motivation for using CAM was to "help their body heal itself", to "boost the immune system" and to "give a sense of control over their treatment".

In qualitative studies on the use of CAM, there are reports on the difficulties and advantages observed by patients who opt for treatment with these methods, such as: i) the tension between the perceived need for restrictive self-discipline and a sense of emancipatory potential, ii) the role of therapists in reconceptualizing the illness, and iii) the complex interaction between self-healing notions and acceptance of individual mortality.

Patients with a history of healing from chronic pathologies describe that the clinical skills that facilitate these processes are: self-confidence, emotional self-management, attention and knowledge. And that three points developed in these processes were: trust, hope, and a sense of self-knowledge.

A Canadian study corroborates these ideas and concludes that although health professionals may not be able to create transformative experiences for patients, they can establish and maintain conditions that support this process.

2. The Voice of Health Professionals on Self-Healing Practices

A study of 55 hospitals in the United States showed that 63% of hospitals consider themselves holistic places. Of these, 80% offer gardens, visitation and meditation rooms or chapels with religious visits when presented in the inpatient history to improve the health experience; as well as color, light, architecture and nature to create more harmonious environments. They also offered self-care classes such as meditation, nutrition and exercise during hospitalization.

Nurses are the group of health professionals who offer the most alternative modalities. In Israel, they use massage, herbal medicine, meditation, touch therapies and prayer with pregnant and parturient women. While in the UK, therapists reported good acceptance of reiki by patients and staff.

However, there are challenges to this integration, as demonstrated by a study in Canada of 875 doctors who rated homeopathy, naturopathy, Feldenkrais, Rolfing, herbal medicine and traditional Chinese medicine as not being effective. In Australia, 664 health professionals classified these practices as potentially harmful, as they were considered to have side effects.

Others such as acupuncture, massage therapy, chiropractic, relaxation therapy, biofeedback are considered safe, effective and indicated in the treatment of chronic or psychosomatic symptoms, but are less accepted for general indications. While esoteric therapies, such as spiritual healing, aromatherapy and reflexology, were seen as relatively safe, but also ineffective.

In the United States, therapists identify important differences from conventional medicine and consider that attitudes and beliefs are the biggest obstacles to this integration, rather than economic or scientific issues.

A study carried out in American Samoa showed that health professionals use and recommend complementary and alternative medicines popular in the United States, such as exercise, diet, prayer, massage and relaxation techniques. But the majority (72%) believe that local and traditional alternative practices in Samoa are detrimental to the patient's quality of life and advise discontinuing their use.

Work with indigenous shamans and their herbs shows that the Western approach focuses essentially on the efficacy of plant chemistry, whereas a shama pays much more attention to relational aspects, which also involves the plants themselves, as a kind of person (a belief shared by all members of the group).

The challenges, on the one hand, are related to the fact that the visibility of integrative and complementary practices is only possible in relation to conventional practices, and, on the other, the notable differences in the logics of operation of allopathic medicine, based on the discourse on disease and symptomatological cure; and complementary and alternative medicine, based on the maintenance of health.

There are proposals for this integration, such as that of doctor Gonzalez (2008), who believes that conventional medicine should be aligned with the idea of returning to a state of health by restoring normal physiology and metabolism.

Currently, when medical students reach the clinical cycle, they only study drugs and high-tech diagnostic and interventional equipment, which will enable them to disrupt the perfect metabolic pathways and physiological systems that they studied in the basic cycle at university.

Thus, through a faithful and comprehensive partnership established between the pharmaceutical industry and the medical services industry, allopathic practice crystallizes in professional life.

What's more, the numerous unnecessary procedures and medications, errors and false diagnoses were the leading cause of death in the United States in 2007, surpassing heart disease and cancer.

For Moritz (2011), scientific research should not be used exclusively to formulate a certain truth, as it is very easy to use studies to manipulate opinions and beliefs. He cites as an example the FDA (Food and Drug Administration) in the United States, which removes 150 drugs a year from the market because of the side effects they cause in many patients. These same drugs have been tested by clinical studies and approved by this supervisory agency in previous years.

For Trudeau (2004), the issue of monitoring medicines and food products is aggravated by the fact that most of the people involved in releasing these products for sale belonged to the companies subjected to the tests and that, therefore, the results would not be impartial.

In Brazil, this complicity is established in the second and third phases of exploratory therapy, when the side effects of the drugs are not yet fully known. Examples include Vioxx® and Celebra®, which were brought to the country as anti-inflammatory drugs with no gastrointestinal effects, but after years of use in millions of patients, have been shown to double the risk of heart attacks and strokes.

The majority of current clinical diagnostic methods for chronic illnesses focus on symptoms and therefore hide or don't treat the causes of these symptoms. Natural therapies that have the knowledge to prevent and cure the most diverse diseases, which are not patentable, are replaced by patentable and therefore profitable synthetic therapies.

Severe cases of illness are subjected to invasive tests and methods that often cause side effects that are worse than the initial symptom, such as chemotherapy. It is considered acceptable and fatal if the patient dies during treatment. However, if a person opts for an alternative treatment and suffers the same end, the patient will be considered reckless and irresponsible, and the doctor will be punished for it.

This is what happened to Danish doctor Kirstine Nolfi[130] in Denmark in 1950, after the death of two patients. She was held responsible by the medical authorities for the deaths of these people and lost her right to practice medicine, despite the fact that the patients' relatives defended her during the trial for encouraging treatment through raw foodism.

Another current example in Brazil was the decision by the Regional Council of Medicine of the State of Rio de Janeiro (Cremeij) in 2012 to send a complaint to the Regional Council of Medicine of the State of São Paulo (Cremesp) against obstetrician Jorge Kuhn. The complaint was prompted by his participation in a television report defending home births.

The Biosaude group has been in the media countless times accused of carrying out dangerous and fraudulent activities. They use the method of bioenergetics (a technique inspired by applied kinesiology), and through muscle tests they detect the cause and indicate the treatment with simple, accessible and natural resources, such as tea, clay and sunbathing.

The same technique criticized by the media is disseminated under the name "Bidigital Ring Test (BDORT)" by the Brazilian Medical Association of Acupuncture, about which there are books and published articles demonstrating the method's effectiveness. But instead of using the tunic to test treatments that are accessible from nature, they use it to prescribe drugs.

The common axis of practices governed by the principles of self-healing is reconnection with the simple and inexpensive resources that nature offers, such as healthy eating, breathing and exercise. These are practices that are always mentioned in academic and media circles, but which are not present in the daily routine of patients and health centers.

That's why these groups shouldn't be seen as enemies of the current health system, and should therefore be fought against. They are positive experiences that could be supported and studied, allowing for a greater understanding of their benefits and limitations.

Discussed and applied in health education systems, they could broaden the limited vision of health professionals who only act on the symptom and help with the current difficult integration between conventional and alternative medicine.

As these practices do not involve patenting, there is no interest from industries and companies, so it is the academic communities that will be the ideal environments for this research to develop. Universities can become the greatest allies of a new awareness, in which allopathic medicines will only be used in the appropriate dose and at the appropriate time.

In Brazil, the guidelines of the National Health Promotion Policy and the National Integrative and Complementary Practices Policy encourage research into health promotion and alternative practices, respectively, by evaluating the efficiency, efficacy, effectiveness and safety of the actions and care provided.

In order for this discussion to be encouraged in universities, it is important to include subjects in health teaching institutions and post-graduate courses focused on this issue.

Two articles with nursing students showed that more than 85% of the students wanted more education on the subject, without necessarily learning the skills to perform these therapies.

This is already becoming a reality in some North American universities that have Integrative Medicine curricula, which aim to integrate the various biopsychosocial aspects, in which the individual's interactions with their family and social environment are studied in order to understand the health-disease process.

3. Paths to Self-Healing

Since childhood, our parents, teachers and society in general have convinced us that our bodies are fragile, especially when the aging process begins to show its first signs.

We are educated to delegate our perceptions and decisions about our bodies to other people, who are considered experts in the functioning of the organism, and so we crowd public health systems for simple symptoms. After a long wait, we are usually medicated, and if we don't receive a prescription, we believe that we have not been treated.

The feeling of not being able to do something for yourself, of not having control over yourself, is one of the most common reasons for physical and mental illness. Most people call this feeling "stress". The idea of vulnerability and insecurity generates fear and triggers profound biochemical changes in the body.

The human body is not designed for illness; on the contrary, it has many programs of its own to maintain a perfect state of balance and to restore itself in the event of disharmony.

The nature of human beings is to be healthy, but it's up to us to establish the conditions necessary for this program to work effectively. It would be simplistic to believe that vitamins, a new drug, an intervention or an alternative medical treatment could remedy the effects of many years of neglect. The body has had to endure a lot of pressure during years of poor nutrition, insufficient sleep and lack of adequate exercise.

Health also disappears when happiness disappears. Any action that takes us away from this purpose is related to failure or to creating obstacles that appear so that we can return to the path of happiness.

The state of health is a reflection of how each person perceives themselves and the world around them, and recovering it doesn't consist of resorting to a quick, magical solution;

on the contrary, it's a process of reconstruction that affects every facet of our lives.

There is an enormous latent healing potential within everyone to restore balance to body, mind and spirit. Utilizing one's own healing powers creates a comforting and permanent space, a continuous sense of satisfaction, and the basis for a creative, prosperous and fulfilling life.

BODY

The microbiological theory of diseases, on which the modern medical system is based, was postulated by the French chemist Louis Pasteur at the end of the 19th century, in which every infectious disease has its cause (etiology) in a microbe with the ability to spread among people, so treatment must seek out the microorganism responsible for each disease in order to determine a way to combat it.

Pasteur, at the end of his life, would have admitted that his fellow countryman and rival Antoine Bĕchamp, a French chemist and biologist, was correct in stating that the ecology of the blood and tissues plays a decisive role in determining whether a disease will manifest itself, demonstrating that if the acid-base balance (pH) of the body is tending towards acidity, the body becomes a favorable environment for destructive microorganisms and the risk of becoming ill increases.

Therefore, illness is a manifestation of a crisis of toxicity in the body, which produces an environment conducive to the multiplication of microbes. Toxins include chemical food additives, environmental contamination, metabolic residues (such as adrenaline released in times of stress) and the toxicity generated by bacteria and fungi that decompose food that has not been assimilated by the digestive system.

In the USA, 95% of patients with Chemical Sensitivity Syndrome who sought complementary therapies were advised to change their diet, looking for products free of chemicals (agrotoxins, preservatives, flavorings, colorings, etc.).

Trudeau (2004) suggests the existence of a network created to generate diseases, in which the population is poisoned by products rich in chemical additives (coloring, flavoring, emulsifiers, monosodium glutamate, etc.), and then uses medicines.

In the same way, the components of nature are perfect when used *as they* are, because they are synergistic. But they start to show side effects or no results when one of their components is used in isolation.

One of the articles demonstrates this by using naturopathy to treat earache in 171 children. They were divided to receive treatment with Naturopathic Herbal Extract Drops (NHED) or anesthetic, with or without amoxicillin (antibiotic). The results were better in the NHED group than in the controls. There were no side effects and antibiotic treatment was not contributory. Herbal extracts are easier to administer and cheaper than antibiotics.

Zago (2005), author of the book "Cancer Has a Cure", describes his successful experience using a natural formula made from aloe vera to cure various diseases. He adds that illness arises when you are not in tune with your inner purpose and reports on his experience in a low-income community combining aloe vera treatment with health education.

The classes talked about the importance of happiness (good thoughts), food (without meat), local herbal medicine and self-sufficient food production through the community garden, reducing costs and improving the quality of food by consuming agrotoxin-free products.

The Alimentagao Viva project, coordinated by Dr. Alberto Gonzalez, works in a similar way in Family Health Programs in cities in the interior of the state of Sao Paulo. Patients undergo a medical consultation and are referred to workshops on the preparation of functional foods, thus being invited and trained to be active agents in their healing process.

Moritz (2011) corroborates these ideas and indicates the following as methods to help restore health: vegetarian and organic food, daily hydration and sunbathing, regular physical exercise, detoxification methods (and the suppression of habits that lead to this process: processed foods, tobacco, alcohol), sleep routine, meditation, breathing exercises and natural therapies (urine therapy, geotherapy, gemmotherapy, autohemotherapy, massage therapy, herbal medicine, radiesthesia and art therapy).

These integrative and complementary practices act in the prevention, promotion, maintenance and recovery of health, centered on the integrality of the individual and humanized care.

A group of 25 patients with a history of trauma received psychotherapy and a complementary modality of their choice (massage, acupuncture, and reiki). Positive changes were observed in four dimensions: interpersonal safety, interpersonal shame of limits, body sensations, and body.

In Canada, 46 cancer patients underwent integrative medicine (conventional combined with complementary) and although there were no significant improvements in quantitative measures, the qualitative conclusions indicated that patients felt encouraged to take an active role in self-care.

MIND

The body-mind divide, based on old, outdated paradigms of human behavior, never really existed. The belief that man is essentially physical today ignores the great role that the mind, feelings and emotions play in our well-being.

The current health system seeks to blame illness for our lack of well-being, insisting on fighting it as if it were an enemy. By focusing attention on the disease, or establishing it as a point of reference and certainty in our lives, we are unable to free ourselves from it, since the disease feeds on our negative thinking, causing a strong immune-depressive state and preventing us from effectively recovering our health.

Every thought and feeling is instantly translated into biochemical substances in the brain and other parts of the body. The endocrine system, a personal and free pharmacy, generates hormones in responsc to our mental experiences. The laboratory we all carry inside can manufacture everything we need and we formulate the recipes ourselves.

These substances include stress hormones (adrenaline, cortisol and cholesterol), which when released into the blood can be life-saving, but which can constantly damage blood vessels and affect our immune system. On the other hand, happiness emotions are manifested with endorphins, serotonin and interleukins, which are substances related to pleasant experiences.

Eight case studies with significant results, according to their authors, were published in Israel and used meditation as a technique to facilitate healing and autonomy, helping to connect with their inner voice and find their purpose in life.

In Austria, a study demonstrated the power of belief over treatment. Half (40) of a group of patients with advanced cancer were treated by reik practitioners and the other half (40) by actors (placebo). Both groups improved, demonstrating that more than the technique, the cure lies in the faith.

Another study with the same purpose was carried out in the UK. 60 patients with arthritis were divided into three groups: control (they received no intervention), they received self-reported distant healing from a healer, and "blind" (they received distant healing but had no knowledge of the treatment). In the end, awareness of receiving distant healing was associated with better results.

Being aware of your role in the healing process has also proven to be a valuable tool. A study in which self-applied reiki was used with patients complaining of pain showed that twelve out of 13 participants experienced an improvement in the frequency, intensity or duration of their pain after three treatments. But it was also observed that 11 of the 13 participants experienced profound changes in their view of themselves, their lives, and their potential for healing and transformation.

In the USA, 24 women who had been sexually abused in childhood were offered self-massage and body therapy. They showed improvement after four weeks of sessions and the results lasted even three months after the intervention.

Another article worked with torture trauma with good preliminary results through Qigong and Tai Chi, which are also techniques that provide a means of involving the body and mind in the process of healing trauma.

Art therapy has also been shown to help in this way. Thirty patients with a history of torture-related trauma were enrolled in a program known as "Healing Images", which uses individually chosen images from digital cameras, which are then shared and discussed within the group.

The program's activities triggered a process of self-expression that allowed participants to value themselves and expand their personal growth. The fundamental advantage was the mutual support and the environment for discussions, reducing physical and psychological isolation.

MIDDLE

Two articles carried out in Brazil noted the importance of social support for patients and their families, relating religion to the treatment of psychosis and drug addiction.

Family members turned to religion as a source of healing, to complement psychiatric treatment, as well as for personal relief and comfort. For young people with psychosis, involvement with religion served to communicate, elaborate and transform their experience with the illness; and sometimes to reduce pathology and improve well-being compared to conventional therapies.

Among evangelical drug addicts, religious resources were the treatment, showing a strong aversion to doctors and pharmacological treatment. A common characteristic of Catholic and Protestant groups is the importance attached to praying and talking to God, described by the subjects as a strong anxiolytic, and a means of controlling drug cravings.

The key aspects of this type of treatment are reception, equal and instant treatment, and acceptance, without judgment. The success of these organizations, then, is not only due to some supernatural aspect, as one might suppose, but also more to the unconditional dedication of human beings to their peers.

A study in China corroborates the importance of this support. It showed that the survival rate of early and mid-stage malignant tumors was significantly better in the group that received systematic anti-cancer education over a 2-year period compared to a group that did not receive this support.

Analysis of the health-disease process shows that health is the result of the ways in which production, work and society are organized in a given historical context, and the biomedical apparatus is unable to modify the broader conditioning factors and determinants of this process, operating a model of attention and care marked, most of the time, by the centrality of symptoms. By redefining health as a sense of physical, psychological and social well-being, the World Health Organization has worked to break this paradigm.

At the same time, we must be vigilant, because we see the environment as a mere backdrop, something external, from which we suffer no interference. Environmental degradation has been negatively influencing the health-disease process.

In Iceland, eight patients were interviewed in a hospital that is in a tranquil setting amidst nature, and described that they felt the place had healing effects, i.e. interfered with their healing process; and that the change in space was crucial in focusing their attention on self-healing and developing a better sense of balance between their minds and bodies.

The complexity of environmental problems calls for measures that go beyond welfare practices, leading to the adoption of transdisciplinary solutions. Among the priorities of the National Health Promotion Policy is the stimulation of a culture of peace and the promotion of sustainable development. These approaches increase the co-responsibility of individuals for their health and help to increase the exercise of citizenship.

FINAL CONSIDERATIONS

Illness needs to stop being seen as a punishment and start being recognized for its true function as a messenger. Illness is a reflection in the physical and emotional body of a disharmony in the choices the individual has made for themselves and imbalances in their interaction with the environment.

In order for healing to occur in a lasting way, we need to be aware that the help we receive to overcome the symptoms of a pathology, whether from conventional or alternative health professionals, should not be associated with delegating responsibility and control over the process of becoming ill to another person.

The practice of self-healing requires a reconnection with oneself, so that the individual can re-evaluate his or her life habits, become aware of the power of his or her thoughts and criticize how he or she is interacting with the social and environmental environment.

By understanding the causes of the loss of health, a new challenge presents itself: to encourage oneself to transform what needs to be renewed, and thus enjoy the conquest over health again.

REFERENCES

ABEL, C.; BUSIA, K. An Exploratory Ethnobotanical Study of the Practice of Herbal Medicine by the Akan Peoples of Ghana. **Alternative Medicine Review**, v. 10, n. 2, p. 112122, 2005.

AIKINS, A.G. Healer shopping in Africa: new evidence from rural-urban qualitative study of Ghanaian diabetes experiences. **BMJ Online First**, v. 331, n. 737, p. 1-7, 2005.

ANANTH, S.; SMITH, K. Optimal Healing Environments. **Explore**, v. 4, n.5, p. 333-334, 2008.

ARYE, E.B. et al. Complementary Medicine in the Primary Care Setting: Results of a Survey of Gender and Cultural Patterns in Israel. **Gender Medicine**, v. 6, n. 2, p. 384-397, 2009.

ASTIN, J.A. Why patients use alternative medicine: results of a national study. **JAMA**, v.279, p. 1548-1553, 1998.

BARRETT, B. et al. What Complementary and Alternative Medicine Practitioners Say About Health and Health Care. **Annals of Family Medicine**, v. 2, n.3, p. 253-259, 2004.

BAZARGAN, M. et al. Correlates of Complementary and Alternative Medicine Utilization in Depressed, Underserved African American and Hispanic Patients in Primary Care Settings. **The Journal of alternative and complementary medicine**, v.14, n.5, p. 537-544, 2008.

BELL, R.A. et al. CAM Use Among Older Adults Age 65 or Older with Hypertension in the United States: General Use and Disease Treatment. **The Journal of alternative and complementary medicine**, v. 12, n.9, p. 903-909, 2006.

BIGNARDI, F.A.C. The transdisciplinary attitude applied to health and sustainability, a multidimensional approach: the importance of meditation. **Terceiro Incluido**, v. 1 n.1, p.1424, 2011.

BIMBAUM, L. Adolescent Aggression and Differentiation of Self: Guided Mindfulness Meditation in the Service of Individuation. The Scientific World Journal, v.5, p. 478-489, 2005

BRAZIL. Ministry of Health. Health Care Secretariat. National Policy for Integrative and Complementary Practices in the SUS (PNPIC-SUS): attitude to expanding access. Brasilia, DF, 2006.

BRAZIL. Ministry of Health. Health Care Secretariat. National Health Promotion Policy (PNPS). Brasilia, DF, 2010.

BRAZIER, A.; COOKE, K.; MORAVAN, V. Using Mixed Methods for Evaluating an Integrative Approach to Cancer Care: A Case Study. **Integrative Cancer Therapies**, v. 7, n.1, p. 5-17, 2008.

BROOM, A. "I'd forgotten about myself in all of this": Discourses of self-healing, positivity and vulnerability in cancer patients' experiences of complementary and alternative medicine. **Journal of Sociology**, v. 45, n.1, p. 71-87, 2009.

BROOM, A.; TOVEY, P. Exploring the Temporal Dimension in Cancer Patients' Experiences of Nonbiomedical Therapeutics. **Qualitative Health Research**, v. 18, n.12, p.1650-1661, 2008.

BROWN, C.M. et al. Patterns of Complementary and Alternative Medicine Use in African Americans. **The Journal of alternative and complementary medicine**, v.13, n.7, p.751-758, 2007.

BRUNING, J. **Are there incurable diseases? : bioenergy and health**. Curitiba: Expoente, 2003.

BRUZOS, G.A.S; KAMIMURALL, H.M.; ROCHALL, S.A.; JORGETTO, T.A.C.; PATRICIO, K. Environment and nursing: their interfaces and insertion in undergraduate teaching. **Saude e Sociedade**, v. 20, n. 2, p. 462-469, 2011.

CHANG, L.H.; WANG, J. Integration of complementary medical treatments with rehabilitation from the perspectives of patients and their caregivers: a qualitative inquiry. **Clin Rehabil**, v. 23, n. 8, p.730-40, 2009.

CHAVES, N. **The health of your eyes: light, darkness and movement**. Rio de Janeiro: Imago, 2002.

CHEUNG, C.K.; WYMAN, J.F.; HALCON, L.L. Use of Complementary and Alternative Therapies in Community-Dwelling Older Adults. **The Journal of alternative and complementary medicine**, v. 13, n. 9, p.997-1006, 2007.

CLARK, C.C. Inner dialogue: A self-healing approach for nurses and clients. **American Journal of Nursing**, v.81, p. 1191-1193, 1981.

COHEN, M.M. et al. The Integration of Complementary Therapies in Australian General Practice: Results of a National Survey. **The Journal of alternative and complementary medicine**, v.11, n.6, p. 995-1004, 2005.

COLLINGE, W.; WENTWORTH, R.; SABO, S. Integrating Complementary Therapies into Community Mental Health Practice: An Exploration. **The Journal of alternative and complementary medicine**, v.11, n.3, p. 569-574, 2005.

CONSTANTINI, A.V.; WIELAND, H.; QVICK, L.I. **The garden of eden, longevity diet.** Fungalbionics series. Germany: Oberlin Verlag, 1998.

CRUS, D.A; WILKINSON, J.M. Reasons for Choosing and Complying with Complementary Health Care: An In-House Study on a South Australian Clinic. **The Journal of alternative and complementary medicine**, v. 11, n.6, p.1107-1112, 2005.

DICKERSO, S.S. et al. Seeking and Managing Hope: Patients' Experiences Using the Internet for Cancer Care. **Oncology Nursing Forum**, v. 33, n.1, p.E8-E17, 2006.

EASTER, A.; WATT, C. It's good to know: How treatment knowledge and belief affect the outcome of distant healing intentionality for arthritis sufferers. **Journal of Psychosomatic Research**, v. 71, p. 86-89, 2011.

FRIES, C.J. Classification of complementary and alternative medical practices. **Canadian Family Physician**, v. 54, p. 1570-1577, 2008.

GARBARINI, N. Heartbeat poetry. **Sci Am**, v.291, n.4, p.13,2004.
GARROW, D.; EGEDE, L.E. National patterns and correlates of complementary and alternative medicine use in adults with diabetes. **The Journal of alternative and complementary medicine**, v.12, n.9, p.895-902, 2006.

GIBSON, P.R.; ELMS, A.N.M.; RUDING, L.A. Perceived Treatment Efficacy for Conventional and Alternative Therapies Reported by Persons with Multiple Chemical Sensitivity. **Environmental Health Perspectives**, v.111, n.12, p.1498-1504, 2003.

GIORDANO, J. et al. Blending the boundaries: steps toward an integration of complementary and alternative medicine into mainstream practice. **J Altern Complement Med**, v.8, n.6, p.897-906, 2002.

GIORDANO, J. et al. Complementary and alternative medicine in mainstream public health: a role for research in fostering integration. **J Altern Complement Med**, v.9, n.3, p.441-5, 2003.

GOODSMITH, L. A look at the "Healing Images" experience. **Torture**, v.17, n. 3, p. 222232, 2007.

GONZALEZ, A.P. Lugar de Mdico ë na Cozinha: cura e saude pela alimentação viva. 6. ed. Sao Paulo: Alaude, 2008.

GOTTSCHLING, S. et al. Use of complementary and alternative medicine in healthy children and children with chronic medical conditions in Germany. **Complementary Therapies in Medicine**, p.1-9, 2011.

GRODIN, M.A. et al. Treating Survivors of Torture and Refugee Trauma: A Preliminary Case Series Using Qigong and T'ai Chi. **The Journal of alternative and complementary medicine**, v.14, n.7, p. 801-806, 2008.

GUNNARSDOTTIR, T.J.; MCALPINE, C.P. The experience of using a combination of complementary therapies: a journey of balance through self-healing. **J Holist Nurs**, v.22, n.2, p.116-32, 2004.

HALCON, L.L. et al. Complementary Therapies and Healing Practices: Faculty/Student Beliefs and Attitudes and the Implications for Nursing Education. **Journal of Professional Nursing**, v. 19, n. 6, p. 387-397, 2003.

HAMRE, H.J. et al. Health costs in anthroposophic therapy users: a two-year prospective cohort study. **BMC Health Services Research**, v. 6, n.65, p. 1-8, 2006.

HASAN, S.S. et al. Reasons, Perceived Efficacy, and Factors Associated with Complementary and Alternative Medicine Use Among Malaysian Patients with HIV/AIDS. **The Journal of alternative and complementary medicine**, v.16, n.11, p. 1171-1176, 2010.

HELYER, L.K. et al. The use of complementary and alternative medicines among patients with locally advanced breast cancer - a descriptive study. **BMC Cancer**. 2006; 6(39): 39-47.
NETP, J.F.R. et al. Common mental disorders and the use of complementary and alternative medicine practices: a population-based study. **J Bras Psiquiatr**, v.57, n.4, p.233239, 2008.

HOLLIDAY, I. Traditional medicines in modern societies: an exploration of integrationist options through East Asian experience. **J Med Philos**, v. 28, n. 3, p. 373-89, 2003.

HONDA, K.; JACOBSON, J.S. Use of complementary and alternative medicine among United States adults: the influences of personality, coping strategies, and social support. **Preventive Medicine**, v. 40, p. 46-53, 2005.

HORI, S. et al. Patterns of complementary and alternative medicine use among outpatients in Tokyo, Japan. BMC Complementary and Alternative Medicine, v.8, n. 14, 2008.

HSU, M.C. et al. Use of Complementary and Alternative Medicine among adult patients for depression in Taiwan. **Journal of Affective Disorders**, v. 111, p. 360-365, 2008.

KRISTOFFERSEN, A.E.; FONNEBO, V.; NORHEIM, A.J. Use of Complementary and Alternative Medicine Among Patients: Classification Criteria Determine Level of Use. **The**

Journal of alternative and complementary medicine, v. 14, n.8, p.911-919, 2008.

KROSCH, S.L. Perceptions and Use of Complementary and Alternative Medicine in American Samoa: A Survey of Health Care Providers. **Hawai'i Medical Journal**, v. 69, n. 3, p. 21-26, 2010.

LAMBERT, T.D. et al. The use of complementary and alternative medicine by patients attending a UK headache clinic. **Complementary Therapies in Medicine**, v.18, p.128-134, 2010.

LENAERTS, M. Substances, relationships and the omnipresence of the body: an overview of Ashdninka ethnomedicine (Western Amazonia). **Journal of Ethnobiology and Ethnomedicine**, v. 2, n. 49, p.1-19, 2006.

LENGACHER, C.A. et al. Frequency of use of complementary and alternative medicine in women with breast cancer. **Oncol Nurs Forum**, v. 29, n.10, p.1445-52, 2002.

LEVIN, J.; TAYLOR, R.J. ; CHATTERSS, L.M. Prevalence and sociodemographic correlates of spiritual healer use: Findings from the National Survey of American Life. **Complementary Therapies in Medicine**, v.19, p. 63-70, 2011.

LORENC, A. et al. The integration of healing into conventional cancer care in the UK. **Complementary Therapies in Clinical Practice**, v.16, p.222-228, 2010.

LUNNY, C.A.; FRASER, S.N. The Use of Complementary and Alternative Medicines Among a Sample of Canadian Menopausal-Aged Women. **Journal of Midwifery & Women's Health**, v. 55, p.335-343, 2010.

MARSH, J. et al. Use of Alternative Medicines by Patients with OA that Adversely Interact with Commonly Prescribed Medications. **Clinical Orthopaedics and Related Research**, v.467, p.2705-2722, 2009.

MATEL, T.L. Contemporary Culture and Alternative Medicines: New Paradigms in Health at the End of the 20th Century. **Rev. Saude Coletiva**, 15(Suplemento), p.145- 176, 2005.

MCKIE, J. A personal conceptualization of healing. **The Australian Journal of Holistic Nursing**, v.10, n. 2, p. 34 -38, 2003.

METCALFE, A. et al. Use of complementary and alternative medicine by those with a chronic disease and the general population - results of a national population based survey. **BMC Complementary and Alternative Medicine**, v. 10, p. 58-63, 2010.

MOLINA, A.I.; LUXARDO, N. Non-conventional medicines in cancer. **Medicina (B Aires)**, v. 65, n.5, p.390-394, 2005.

MORITZ, A. **Los Secretos Eternos de la Salud**. 8. ed. Barcelona: Obelisco, 2011.

MULKINS, A.L.; MORSE, J.M.; BEST, A. Complementary Therapy Use in HIV/AIDS. **Can J Public Health**, v. 93, n.3, p. 308-312, 2002.

MULKINS, A.L.; VERHOEF, M.J. Supporting the Transformative Process: Experiences of Cancer Patients Receiving Integrative Care. **Integrative Cancer Therapies**, v.3, n.3, p.230237, 2004.

NASCIMENTO, M.C. De panacdia mystica a especialidade medica: a acupuntura na vista da imprensa escrita. **Hist Cienc Saude Manguinhos**, v. 5, n. 1, p. 99-113, 1998.

NETO, J.F.R.; FARIA, A.A.; FIGUEIREDO, M.F.S. Prevalence of the use of homeopathy by the population of the city of Montes Claros, Minas Gerais, Brazil. **Rev Assoc Med Bras**, v.127, n.6, p.329-334, 2009.

NGUYEN, L.T. et al. Use of Complementary and Alternative Medicine and Self-Rated Health Status: Results from a National Survey. **J Gen Intern Med**, v. 26. n. 4, p.399-404, 2010.

NOLFI, K. **Los Alimentos Vivos: Mis experiencias com los alimentos vivos**. Palma Mallorca: Coleccion Higiene Vital, 1993.

O'BRIEN K. Complementary and alternative medicine: the move into mainstream health care. Clin Exp Optom, v.87, n.2, p.110-20, 2004.

OLIVEIRA, E.C.M.; POLES, K. Beliefs of patients with chronic wounds: a discursive analysis. **REME**, v.10, n.4, p.354-360, 2006.

OMURA, Y. **The practice of the bioenergetic ring test: BDORT**. Sao Paulo: Brazilian Medical Association of Acupuncture, 2000.

OZTEKIN, D.S. et al. Nursing Students' Willingness to Use Complementary and Alternative Therapies for Cancer Patients: Istanbul Survey. **Tohoku J. Exp. Med**, v. 211, n.1, p. 49-61, 2007.

POHL, G. et al. "Laying on of hands" improves well-being in patients with advanced cancer. **Support Care Cancer**, v. 15, p.143-151, 2007.

PORTER, M. et al. Changing patterns of CAM use among prostate cancer patients two years after diagnosis: Reasons for maintenance or discontinuation. **Complementary Therapies in Medicine**, v. 16, p.318-324, 2008.

PRICE, C. Dissociation reduction in body therapy during sexual abuse recovery. **Complement Ther Clin Pract**, v.13, n.2, p.116-128, 2007.

QUANDT, S.A. et al. Use of Complementary and Alternative Medicine By Persons With Arthritis: Results of the National Health Interview Survey. **Arthritis & Rheumatism (Arthritis Care & Research)**, v.53, n.5, p.748-755, 2005.

QUINN, J.F. The self as healer: Reflections from a nurse's journey. **AACN Clinical Issues**, v. 11, n.1, p.17-26, 2000.

RAUSCH, S.M. et al. Complementary and alternative medicine: use and disclosure in radiation oncology community practice. **Support Care Cancer**, v.19, p. 521-529, 2011.

REDKO, C. Religious Construction of a First Episode of Psychosis in Urban Brazil. **Transcultural Psychiatry**, v. 40, n.4, p.507-530, 2003.

REICH, W. **A. Cancer Biopathy**. Sao Paulo: Martins Fontes, 2009.

REYES, O.C.A.; RODRIGUEZ, M.; MARKIDES, K.S. The Role of Spirituality Healing with Perceptions of the Medical Encounter among Latinos. **J Gen Intern Med**, v. 24, n.3, p. 542547, 2009.

ROBB, W.J.W. Self Healing: A Concept Analysis. **Nursing Forum**, v. 41, n. 2, april/june 2006.

ROLNIAK, S. et al. Complementary and Alternative Medicine Use Among Urban ED Patients: Prevalence and Patterns. **Journal of Emergency Nursing**, v. 30, n.4, p.318-324, 2004.

ROSS, L.E. et al. Prayer and Self-Reported Health Among Cancer Survivors in the United States, National Health Interview Survey, 2002. **The Journal of alternative and complementary medicine**, v.14, n.8, p.931-938, 2008.

ROSSI, P. et al. Use of Complementary and Alternative Medicine by PatientsWith Chronic Tension Type Headache: Results of a Headache Clinic Survey. **Headache**, v. 46, p. 622-631, 2006.

SAKURAGI, S.; SUGIYAMA, Y.; TAKEUCHI, K. Effects of laughing and weeping on mood and heart rate variability. **J Physiol Anthropol Appl Human Sci**, v21, n.3, p.159-65, 2002.

SALVETTI, M.G. et al. Self-efficacy and depressive symptoms in patients with chronic pain. **Rev. Psiq. Clin**, v.34, n. 3, p. 111-117, 2007.

SAMUELS, N. et al. Use of and attitudes toward complementary and alternative medicine among nurse-midwives in Israel. **American Journal of Obstetrics & Gynecology**, v.203, n.341, p. e1-7, 2010.

SANCHEZ, Z.M.; NAPPO, S.A. Religious treatments for drug addiction: An exploratory study in Brazil. **Social Science & Medicine**, v.67, p. 638-646, 2008.

SAQUIB, J. et al. Classification of CAM Use and Its Correlates in Patients With Early-Stage Breast Cancer. **Integrative Cancer Therapies**, v.10, n.2, p.138-147, 2011.

SARREL, E.M.; COHEN, H.A.; KAHAN, E. Naturopathic Treatment for Ear Pain in Children. **Pediatrics**, v. 111, n.5, p. e574-e579, 2003.

SCOTT, J.G. et al. Understanding Healing Relationships in Primary Care. **Ann Fam Med**, v.6, n.4, p. 315-322, 2008.

SHORO, S.A. Complementary and alternative medicine (CAM) among hospitalized patients: Reported use of CAM and reasons for use, CAM preferred during hospitalization, and the socio-demographic determinants of CAM users. **Complementary Therapies in Clinical Practice**, v. 17, p.199-205, 2011.

SIBINGA, S.E.M. et al. Parent-pediatrician communication about complementary and alternative medicine use for children. **Clin Pediatr (Phila)**, v.43, n.4, p. 367-73, 2004.

SMITH, B.W. et al. Who is willing to use complementary and alternative medicine? **Explore**, v. 4, n. 6, p. 359-367, 2008.

SMITH, J.M. **Roleta Genetica-documented health risks of transgenic foods**. Sao Paulo: Editora Joao de Barro, 2009.

SOINTU, E. The search for wellbeing in alternative and complementary health practices. **Sociology of Health & Illness**, v. 28, n.3, p.330-349, 2006.

SOO, I. et al. Use of Complementary and Alternative Medical Therapies in a Pediatric Neurology Clinic. **The Canadian Journal of Neurological Sciences**, v.32, n.4, p.524-528, 2005.

SUTHERLAND, E.G. et al. An HMO-Based Prospective Pilot Study of Energy Medicine for Chronic Headaches: Whole-Person Outcomes Point to the Need for New Instrumentation. **The Journal of alternative and complementary medicine**, v. 15, n.8, p.819-826, 2009.

TRUDEAU, K. **Natural Cures: "They" Don't Want You to Know About**. USA: Alliance Publishing Group, 2004.

UPCHURCH, D.M.; CHYU, L. Use of complementary and alternative medicine among American women. **Women's Health Issues**, v.15, p.5-13, 2005.

VANDECREEK, L. et al. Religious and Nonreligious Coping Methods Among Persons With Rheumatoid Arthritis. **Arthritis & Rheumatism (Arthritis Care & Research)**, v.51, n.1, p.49-55, 2004.

VENTEGODT, S.; CLAUSEN, B.; MERRICK, J. Clinical Holistic Medicine: The Case Story of Anna. III. Rehabilitation of Philosophy of Life During Holistic Existential Therapy for Childhood Sexual Abuse. **The Scientific World Journal**, v. 6, p.2080-2091, 2006.

VENTEGODT, S.; KANDEL, I.; MERRICK, J. Clinical Holistic Medicine (Mindful Short-Term Psychodynamic Psychotherapy Complimented with Bodywork) in the Treatment of Schizophrenia (ICD10-F20/DSM-IV Code 295) and Other Psychotic Mental Diseases. **The Scientific World Journal**, v.7, p. 1987-2008, 2007.

VENTEGODT, S.; MERRICK, J. Clinical Holistic Medicine: The Patient with Multiple Diseases. **The Scientific World Journal**, v.5, p.324-339, 2005.

VENTEGODT, S.; MERRICK, J. The Life Mission Theory IV. Theory on Child Development . **The Scientific World Journal**, v. 3, p.1294-1301, 2003.

VENTEGODT, S. et al. Clinical Holistic Medicine: A Pilot Study on HIV and Quality of Life and a Suggested Cure for HIV and AIDS. **The Scientific World Journal**, v. 4, p.264-272, 2004.

VENTEGODT, S. et al. Clinical Holistic Medicine: Holistic Sexology and Treatment of Vulvodynia Through Existential Therapy and Acceptance Through Touch. **The Scientific World Journal**, v. 4, p. 571-580, 2004.

VENTEGODT, S. et al. Clinical Holistic Medicine (Mindful, Short-Term Psychodynamic Psychotherapy Complemented with Bodywork) Improves Quality of Life, Health, and Ability by Induction of Antonovsky- Salutogenesis. **The Scientific World Journal**, v.7, p.317-323, 2007.

VENTEGODT, S. et al. Clinical Holistic Medicine (Mindful, Short-Term Psychodynamic Psychotherapy Complemented with Bodywork) in the Treatment of Experienced Impaired Sexual Functioning. **The Scientific World Journal**, v. 7, p. 324-329, 2007.

VENTEGODT, S. et al. Clinical Holistic Medicine (Mindful, Short-Term Psychodynamic Psychotherapy Complemented with Bodywork) in the Treatment of Experienced Mental Illness. **The Scientific World Journal**, v. 7, p.306-309, 2007.

VENTEGODT, S. et al. Clinical Holistic Medicine: Problems in Sex and Living Together. **The Scientific World Journal**, v. 4, p.562-570, 2004.

VENTEGODT, S. et al. Self-Reported Low Self-Esteem. Intervention and Follow-Up in a Clinical Setting. **The Scientific World Journal**, v.7, 2007.

VENTEGODT, S. et al. The Life Mission Theory VI. A Theory for the Human Character: Healing with Holistic Medicine Through Recovery of Character and Purpose of Life. **The Scientific World Journal**, v. 4, p. 859-880, 2004.

WOLSKO, P.M. et al. Use of Mind-Body Medical Therapies Results of a National Survey. **J Gen Intern Med**, v.19, p.43-50, 2004.

XIAOMEI, H.; JINGCHUAN, F. The Effect of a Complex Healing Treatment on 2-Year Survival Rate of Patients With Malignant Tumors. **Integrative Cancer Therapies**, v.7, n.1, p.18-23, 2008.

YUN, A.J.; LEE, P.Y.; BAZAR, K.A. Paradoxical strategy for treating chronic diseases where the therapeutic effect is derived from compensatory response rather than drug effect. **Med Hypotheses**, 2004.

YUN, A.J. et al. The dynamic range of biologic functions and variation of many environmental cues may be declining in the modern age: implications for diseases and therapeutics. **Medical Hypotheses**, v.65, p.173-178, 2005.

ZAGO, F.R. **Cancer has a Cure**. 34 ed. Petropolis: Editora Vozes, 2005.

ZHANG, X. Integration of traditional and complementary medicine into national health care systems. **J Manipulative Physiol Ther**, v.23, n. 2, p. 139-40, 2000.

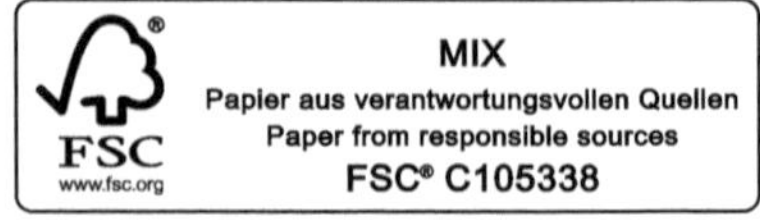

Printed by Books on Demand GmbH, Norderstedt / Germany